THIS NOTEBOOK BELONGS TO:

Made in the USA
Monee, IL
02 December 2020

50521944R00066